HOW TO BANISH COLDS AND INFLUENZA

Medical research workers have frequently shown that none of the much-advertised remedies for the common cold and influenza has the slightest effect on the patient's speed of recovery. But these ailments may be overcome completely and permanently when the causes are treated by the Nature Cure methods explained in this book.

By the same author
OVERCOMING ANAEMIA

How to Banish Colds and Influenza

George J. Hall N.D., D.O.

THORSONS PUBLISHERS LIMITED
Wellingborough, Northamptonshire

First published 1957
Second Edition, revised and reset, 1973
Third Impression 1982

ISBN 0 7225 0218 4

Printed and bound in Great Britain by
Richard Clay (The Chaucer Press) Ltd.,
Bungay, Suffolk.

Contents

Preface to Second Impression

SINCE THIS BOOK was first published a great deal of medical research has been carried out on the subject of colds and influenza. The Common Cold Research Unit at Salisbury has been working since 1946 and it is claimed that a number of viruses which cause colds have been identified.

However, as Dr. Louis Lasagna, Associate Professor, Johns Hopkins Medical School points out (*Reader's Digest*, October, 1963) 'volunteers at the Common Cold Research Unit at Salisbury were given a hot bath, after which they stood for half an hour in wet bathing suits in a draughty corridor, and then wore wet socks. Others, sent on tiring walks in icy rain, returned to their quarters without heat. No colds developed. Even a dose of cold virus given to these hardy souls failed to induce colds'. Medical 'progress' in the U.S.A. appears to be no less disappointing. Under the heading, 'Doubts Over Influenza Vaccine – Does Mass Use Do Any Good?' *Medical News* (22 November, 1963) reported that 'three senior U.S. Public Health Service doctors expressed doubts about the value of mass influenza immunisation programmes. Their case rests upon the fact that excess deaths from influenza and pneumonia reached a figure of 12,000 during last February, March and April, despite the 42 million doses of influenza vaccine used.' It was reported that an epidemiologist, addressing the American Public Health Association, questioned whether results justified the expense of further mass immunisation.

There can be no denying that the situation, in so far as the sufferer is concerned, remains unchanged. It is not surprising therefore to find that the demand for information on the Nature Cure solution to the problem of colds and influenza continues to increase.

February, 1964   G.J.H.

Introduction

'CURES' FOR THE common cold are legion. The reason being, of course, that not one of them does 'cure'. Sufferers go from one remedy to the next — and from one cold to the next!

Old ideas like 'sweat it out', 'work it off', 'kill it', 'feed it', 'drown it', etc., have about as much logic behind them as medical methods of antibiotic therapy, calcium therapy and vaccination. Each of them is a shot in the dark with little more than wishful thinking to back it up.

Effective treatment can only follow a clear understanding of the nature of the disease, and it is the Nature Cure school alone that has offered a logical explanation for the disease and, therefore, a rational and truly effective treatment.

A great deal of time and money has been, and is being, spent on medical research to find 'the cause' of the common cold. Research workers are rummaging through the washings from people's noses, where one would expect the find the *result* of a cold, but not its cause.

However, it has been decided that the cause must be some sort of germ — a virus, in fact — and the search must go on.

Many years ago the cause of influenza was thought to be a germ, which was duly named the *bacillus influenzae*, but no medical man believes this now.

We are not being facetious when we say that to find the cause of both the common cold and influenza one must look beyond one's nose.

Those who practice orthodox medicine are inclined to assume that if they do not know the answer to ill-health, then it is not known; but increasing numbers of sick people are turning to Nature Cure and finding the answer to their health problems.

It is the purpose of this book to make clear to those who have little or no knowledge of the philosophy and practice of Nature Cure the nature of the common cold, its successful prevention and its treatment.

'The proof of the pudding is in the eating', and no-one can judge Nature Cure without the experience of participation. We can only say that those who put it to the test will not be disappointed.

I.
Defining a Cold

ONE OF THE first medically-fostered fallacies that we must expose is the idea that a cold is an entity. It is said that a person 'catches a cold', that he wishes to 'get rid of a cold', and that he is in search of 'a cure for a cold'.

This idea leads to the belief in 'cures' for 'diseases' without consideration of persons. The notion that 'disease' can be kept in a laboratory and that a 'cure' can be produced in a test-tube is not acceptable to the Nature Cure school of thought, but this will be explained later in the book.

The point which has to be made at this stage, however, is that what is usually called 'a disease' is, in fact, a *bodily condition*; it is not something that *attacks* the body. Disease is made evident by the appearance of a number of signs and symptoms, and the name given to it depends upon the combination of symptoms manifest in any particular case.

A cold, then, is a bodily condition which shows certain characteristic symptoms, and it is important to consider these symptoms if we are to have a clear understanding of our subject.

The streaming nose, resulting from inflammation of the upper air passages, is generally considered to be an independent affection and is named *a cold*, or *acute coryza*; but this is not necessarily the case. The first symptoms of measles are those of a severe cold, with streaming nose and eyes, and intense wretchedness. The symptoms of hay-fever are those of an unusually obstinate or persistently recurrent cold, and the main difference between a cold and influenza is in the severity of the symptoms. Acute coryza is also a common symptom of whooping-cough and a number of other diseases.

Again, although the above-mentioned diseases have the common symptom of acute coryza, each case will have its own variation in one respect or another, for, as has been truly said, 'there are as many diseases as there are human beings'.

This may appear to make our subject more difficult to follow but, as will be seen later, it actually simplifies the problem of treatment. The point to be remembered here is that we are not considering different *diseases* but different *individuals* who show similar, though not necessarily identical, symptoms.

The early sumptoms of a developing cold are a feeling of chilliness, slight headache and frequent sneezing. There is usually a slight rise in temperature, and, in severe cases, there are pains in the back and legs. The mucous membrane that lines the nose becomes congested and swollen, causing the nostrils to become 'stopped up', and so the patient has to breath through the mouth. Then, a thin, clear nasal secretion begins to flow, and this irritates the edges of the nostrils and the upper lip, making them red and sore.

The mucous membranes of the tear-ducts become inflamed, causing the eyes to weep. The throat, too, becomes inflamed, with consequent redness and soreness, and sometimes, it becomes difficult to swallow. When the larynx is involved, the voice becomes husky or is even lost. Bronchitis and cough may follow.

A small tube (the Eustachian tube) connects the throat with the ear, and when this becomes inflamed there may be ear-ache or impairment of hearing.

The lining membrane of the sinuses also are continuous with those of the nose and throat, and so sinusitis is a common extension of this inflammatory process.

It should be realized that such names as pharyngitis, laryngitis, bronchitis, rhinitis, stomatitis, sinusitis, blepharitis, etc., merely indicate the site of inflammation and do not constitute distinct 'diseases'.

Usually, within from twenty-four to forty-eight hours, the nasal secretion becomes more profuse, and as the swelling of the mucous membrane subsides the patient gradually becomes able to breathe through his nostrils. Within four or five days most of the symptoms disappear, with the exception of the increased discharge of thick, tenacious mucus from all the membranes involved.

The period of elimination of mucus will vary with individuals; in some, a more or less abrupt ending occurs after about a week, and in others a chronic catarrh of the nose, throat or bronchi continues until the next cold comes along.

The frequency of colds varies also, for whilst to some people a cold is an occasional inconvenience, to others it is but a link in a chain of miserable illness that lasts more or less the whole year through.

To define a cold, then, in terms of signs and symptoms may be useful for the purpose of making medical records, but it does not help those who are trying to understand the nature of disease. Nothing could be more confusing than to rename a disease because of the appearance of one or two additional symptoms.

Symptoms, as we have said, are merely indications of the functioning condition of the body. What we are really concerned with is the change in the bodily condition which brings about the symptoms.

2.
The Relationship of Health and Disease

THAT NATURAL LAW governs all life is indisputable. To attempt the evasion of natural law is to court disaster. Our bodies have certain requirements which are essential for the efficient functioning of the organism, and to deny the body those requirements must mean malfunctioning. Similarly, certain conditions are detrimental to the efficient functioning of the organism, and their avoidance is essential to health.

Again, the restoration of normality (health) to an ill-functioning (diseased) organism demands nothing less than the supply of the necessary ingredients of health and the removal of the causes of ill-health.

Just as unwholesome foods may be 'doctored' and given the appearance of freshness, and the colour, odour and flavour of natural, wholesome foods, so, too, can the human body be doctored and given *the appearance* of freedom from disease. But when the symptoms of disease are *suppressed*, health is in no way restored; indeed, very frequently, the level of health is still further reduced because the agents used to erase the symptoms are usually damaging to the organism. Poisonous drugs, for instance, are no less poisonous when administered to the sick than they are to the healthy. Poisons create ill-health, and they cannot therefore restore good health.

Here, then, is the Nature Cure objection to the practice of medicine. By treating 'diseases' – that is, the removal of symptoms without concern for causes – natural law is violated and consequently no provision is made for the restoration of true health.

The Nature Cure philosophy and practice is founded solidly on well-proved physiological and biological facts, and a short description of the basic principles of health and disease will enable the reader to follow the logic of the Nature Cure attitude towards the common cold.

The body requires certain substances for growth, repair and energy output. These are obtained from air, water, sunshine and the foods we eat. The body discards the unwanted portions of these substances and also the waste products which result from the chemical and physiological transformation of matter within the body.

These processes of absorption, assimilation and elimination are carried out by the innate intelligence of the body without any conscious effort on our part. Certain other factors, however, do have a profound influence upon these processes, including postural and other habits, physical exertion, emotion, thoughts, etc. So long as the body is unhindered, perfect harmony of function results, and this condition is known as health.

Ill-health begins long before the symptoms of disease appear. It commences when the body is deprived of the necessary nutrients; when elimination lags behind the body's encumbrance with morbid matter (toxins); when the body is sapped of its vitality and, therefore, rendered incapable of efficient function.

When the symptoms of disease do appear, they vary according to the combination of causative factors involved, and, as previously stated, the combinations may vary from one individual to another. However, it is agreed that there are similar combinations of symptoms classified as the common cold, influenza, etc., and to discuss these we must find a factor which is common to all such cases. This factor is toxaemia — blood-saturation with toxic substances.

3.
Toxaemia

THE BLOOD ALWAYS carries toxins. One of the functions of the blood — equal in importance to that of delivering nutriment to the tissue-cells — is that of transporting toxins to the eliminative organs (skin, lungs, kidneys, bowel).

Toxaemia is the condition which arises when the body's eliminative effort becomes inadequate and the toxin content of the blood rises considerably above the normal level. This may result from an excessive toxin production, or from failure of the eliminative organs, or both..

These toxic substances are many and varied, although their effect upon the organism is the same — poisoning. Carbonic acid is a poisonous waste product of the process of oxidation which is constantly taking place in the tissues; it is eliminated, mainly, by the lungs. Increased oxidation means, therefore, an increase of carbonic acid, but, normally, the body can cope with the situation by increasing the rate of respiration. In other words, the lungs eliminate faster to keep the blood-level normal.

Other substances for elimination include all the various end-products of metabolism, the waste from spent tissue-cells and secretions, and toxic substances that have been absorbed into the body from outside. Among the latter group may be included drugs and other medicines (including vaccines and sera), nicotine and other substances from tobacco, the products of decomposition and fermentation from within an unhealthy digestive tract, alcohol, chemicals that have been added to food (such as soil fertilizers, insecticides, preservatives, dyes, bleaches, artificial flavours, conditioners, extenders, etc.), and all the food elements that are taken in excess of body requirements.

It is commonly supposed that if a particular food element is 'good for you' then *a lot of it* must be even better for you. Such is not the case, however. Far too often people overfeed themselves on supplementary vitamins (frequently synthetic), energy foods, so-called, such as glucose, body-building proteins, etc. Admittedly, the body can store a small proportion of certain substances, but for the most part these excesses constitute toxins and throw added work upon the eliminative organs.

Despite the fact that modern civilized living (especially eating!) had greatly increased our toxic load, the body still finds ways and means of overcoming the dangers. Of course, there is a limit to the body's capacity for adaptation, and disease and death are the final results of an out-of-hand toxaemia.

The healthy eliminative organs are at work more or less constantly. Kidney function brings about a continuous drain of excess water from the blood, and dissolved in this water are various toxic substances including certain acids, for the blood and tissues will not tolerate an acid medium. Many medicines are disposed of through this channel (although not without first adding to the body's burden of toxins) and any excess of certain vitamins is also 'poured down the drain' in this way.

The skin, which is sometimes called the third kidney, similarly excretes toxic matter in solution, but its function is governed partly by the body's heat regulating mechanism. This is because loss of moisture by evaporation from the surface of the skin reduces body temperature considerably and this is not always desirable.

The main function of the bowel is, of course, to carry away

the food-residue after completion of the digestive processes. This waste at no time enters the blood and, therefore, is not 'eliminated' as a blood-toxin. In certain cases of digestive disorder, the poisonous products of fermentation and decomposition may be absorbed into the blood and then require to be excreted again. Sometimes, however, the bowel is used for the excretion of toxic matter — notably, certain drugs. The lungs have been mentioned already as important excretory organs, for carbonic acid in particular.

This wonderful arrangement of toxin-disposal appears even more remarkable when we realize that when one eliminative organ suffers inhibited function another will compensate, at least in part, either temporarily or permanently. In the event of the total eliminative effort proving to be inadequate, other organs or tissues may be brought into action as auxiliaries.

Here, then, is the situation. The blood and other tissue fluids are continuously receiving and throwing off toxins, and a state of balance is generally maintained through the body's power of adaptability, even when the toxin load is unusually heavy.

But what is likely to happen if elimination is checked? Obviously, toxaemia must result, and, although the body can learn to tolerate a certain degree of toxaemia, there comes a time when urgent action is necessary to reduce the load to a lower and less damaging level. When this urgent action is taken, then the symptoms which arise are said to be those of acute disease.

4.
Acute Disease

MORE OR LESS violent eliminative crises may take any number of forms.

The vitality of the organism, the nature of the toxins requiring elimination, the particular organs involved in the crisis, the exciting cause of the crisis, and many other factors will predetermine the form of action and its intensity. The symptom of diarrhoea indicates that the intestinal tract is playing its part in the eliminative effort. The skin may act by increased perspiration or by the development of an eruption. Respiration may become faster and shallower. The kidneys may throw off a hyper-acid urine, but this is not usually detectable except through chemical tests. In some cases, the mucous membranes of the body play a part in the process of elimination, and the resulting conditions have been classified as influenza, colds, measles, etc. As we have emphasised, already, however, these are not distinct 'diseases', but only variations of the common, acute disease of toxin elimination.

The confusing medical procedure of giving a separate name to every slight variation in the process of acute disease is absolutely pointless for our purpose, and when this is fully realized much of the fear of acute disease will be dispelled.

In 1955, the national newspapers reported that 'a mystery epidemic that has baffled the country's top medical specialists is hitting London'. In three weeks, two hundred and fifty children were 'attacked' by an *unknown* germ.

The germ that could not be found was *thought to be* a highly infectious virus, but it was reported that consultants at a London hospital failed to identify it. To people unfamiliar with medical scaremongering, this would seem a matter for serious concern and urgent action. It is by such scaremongering that the people are brought to (the medical) heel, and thereby cajoled into submitting to all manner of unwholesome injections, subscribing to research funds, and accepting the opinion of 'top medical specialists' as the last word.

The 'new disease' manifested symptoms similar to those which occur in many childish ailments — sore throat, listlessness, and slight swelling of the glands of the throat — but it did not fit in absolutely with any of the usual patterns of acute disease. However, all the children recovered health with no other treatment than rest in bed for forty-eight hours.

It is important to appreciate the unity of the acute reactions observed during eliminative crises, and also to realise that they are designed for the purpose of tissue cleansing. Acute disease is not an 'attack' upon the body, it is *action* on the part of the body. By such an intense action the body is enabled is to relieve itself of sufficient toxic matter to obviate immediate dangers. In some cases a complete cleansing takes place, but this point will be explained later.

The exciting causes of an acute eliminative crisis are countless, but the direct effect of them all upon the body is enervation; enervation, by impeding normal tissue activity, checks elimination. Once elimination is slowed down an accumulation of morbid matter within the tissue fluids soon develops and an eliminative crisis becomes inevitable. Enervation means, of course, loss of vigour, and its causes, as stated previously, are countless. We expend energy with our every move — mental and physical — but in the normal way this expenditure is made good by mental and physical rest (which includes sleep) and proper nourishment. The greater the expenditure of energy, the greater is the need for rest. When the drain on vitality exceeds its regeneration, then enervation is the result.

Human beings have found very many ways of expending energy excessively. To name a few, there are excesses of work, play, eating, worry, anxiety, anger and stimulation with tobacco, alcohol, drugs, etc.

This explains the incidence of epidemic diseases. Large numbers of people whose mode of living is similar, become enervated at much the same time, due to the same causes, and develop similar acute reactions.

Christmastide is a favourite time for overeating (mainly bad mixtures of the wrong foods), overdrinking (often of strong alcoholics), heavy smoking, late nights, over-excitement, foul atmospheres, etc., and it is generally followed by a spate of ill-health.

Colds and influenza are generally considered to be winter ailments, but they do, in fact, occur at all times of the year.

Every sufferer tries to pin down the reason for his ailment to one specific cause, but he only looks back a day or two. Consequently, the blame is laid on to 'a draught on the neck, at a friend's house', 'letting in the night air on an autumn night', 'casting a clout before May is out', 'running to the corner-shop without a hat', 'being caught in the rain' — or one of a million other factors!

It is significant that the sufferer always seeks the cause outside of himself. He never suspects that *he* may be the brewer of his own discomfort. But, then, his medical advisers will tell him that he 'probably picked up a germ', or they will strive in some other way to relieve the patient of his own responsibilities.

Enervation and toxaemia, then, are the causes of acute disease in general, but, here, we are concerned particularly with the common cold and influenza, so let us turn to the characteristic symptoms which are considered to be one of the major causes of industrial absenteeism.

5.
The Respiratory Symptoms

THE MUCOUS MEMBRANE that lines the respiratory tract is exceedingly sensitive to irritation. It is essential that it should be if if it is to protect the organism against respiratory obstruction. The nose, throat, bronchi and lungs are constantly at work collecting and expelling foreign matter, such as dust, by means of the constant flow of mucus and by such reflex actions as sneezing, swallowing and coughing.

The normal physiological action taken by mucous-cells under irritation is increased function, which means an increased flow of mucus. In certain instances, irritation may be sufficiently severe to condition the cells to an increased flow even long after the irritant has been removed.

Numerous dusts and chemicals (including gases) can induce a coryza as is seen in the common cold, but, of course, without giving rise to any other symptoms. Even long-continued exposure to a cold wind may cause running of the nose.

This sensitivity to irritation applies equally to irritation from within as from without. If the blood and other tissue fluids carry substances of an irritant nature, then a similar condition of hyper-secretion results. Certain drugs, such as potassium iodide, have been found guilty in this respect, but we are more concerned with the irritant effect of *toxaemia* as already defined.

Through this tissue-cell sensitivity, the toxic organism,

demanding a greater eliminative effort, will make use of the mucous membranes as auxiliaries to the normal eliminative organs.

When the flow of mucus is more or less continually excessive, the condition is known as *chronic* catarrh, whether this be of the nose (nasal catarrh), of the throat (catarrhal pharyngitis), or of the windpipes (bronchial catarrh). The catarrh which is of sudden onset is variously called acute coryza, acute pharyngitis, acute bronchitis, etc.

It must be remembered that the toxins that are eliminated in the form of catarrh are systemic poisons and they are therefore damaging to tissue cells.

Cellular degeneration is the ultimate outcome of any toxic influence, and that is why the organism strives to free itself as speedily as possible. But if the mucous membranes are employed permanently as eliminators they will suffer from this toxic influence. Here lies the foundation of the many complications, or extensions, of chronic catarrh. The degenerative change that takes place as the result of chronic poisoning will, naturally, depend upon the influence of the particular toxin (or toxins) involved in each case. These tissues will also suffer from exhaustion.

As a result of chronic catarrhal inflammation the vascular nasal tissues become permanently distended and the mucous-cells become swollen from absorption of transuded lymph. The surface cells proliferate, desquamate and degenerate. This condition is frequently associated with exostosis (outgrowths of bone) and ecchondroses (outgrowths of cartilage) of the nasal septum and other parts of the nose, and polypi are common. Nasal obstruction leads to mouth breathing and further trouble.

Here, too, is a site for bacterial *activity*. The actual *presence* of bacteria is of little significance, for, as is now well known, most pathogenic organisms, so-called, may be present in the nose and throat of healthy people. Indeed, it would be impossible to live life without coming into contact with these micro-organisms. They are more or less everywhere, awaiting a job of work to do.

Their function throughout nature, and not simply in relation to human disease, is the breaking down of complicated organic substances into simpler compounds or elements. But for their action the decomposition of vegetable and animal waste would be impossible, and the cycle of life would be broken. The gardener realizes this when he encourages bacterial growth in his compost heap, for he desires that his refuse be broken down to the simple substances necessary for plant growth. But it is the dead, dying and diseased animal and vegetable matter that is broken down, not healthy, living tissues. The tissues of a marrow plant, or a mushroom, will *thrive* on a compost heap which is teeming with bacteria.

The living human intestine swarms with bacteria whose purpose it is to break down some of the complex substances eaten by us as food. The less complex substances produced by bacterial activity, which we are able to absorb and utilize, include certain vitamins which would not otherwise be available to us.

Wherever human tissues are found to be breaking down, so, too, are we likely to find bacterial scavengers of one sort or another. The more devitalized the state of the tissues, the greater will be bacterial activity and proliferation.

No less than human beings, every type of micro-organism has its own particular requirements for growth and multiplication, and since the human body can supply a number of different media for bacterial growth, it is to be expected that each strain will show preference for the conditions best suited to its requirements.

It was the association of definite microbic types with certain disease states which led to the widely accepted view that 'germs cause disease'. Whilst the naturopath agrees that these organisms may throw off waste products of their own which are toxic to the human organism, he insists that it is the disease state which exists first, and so provides the 'soil' for bacterial growth.

There is, of course, ample evidence to show that this view is justified. The healthy throat may harbour the germs commonly associated with such 'diseases' as diptheria, influenza, pneumonia, scarlet fever, etc., without the appearance of any sign of disease. On the other hand, disease can, and frequently does, exist without the presence of the germ.

The mucous membranes of a toxaemic person may provide the ideal organic substance, or 'soil', for a certain strain of micro-organisms, but the 'disease' already exists. Bacterial infection is secondary.

The old idea that the germ *is* the disease has led to a situation in which the whole civilized world is living in a constant dread of these 'unseen enemies of man'. People have become afraid of social contact, afraid even of shaking hands with their friends, lest they 'pick up a germ'. Useless antiseptics are used on every occasion, and the chemical and biological manufacturers are alive to the possibilities of extending the use of this heaven-sent, money-circulating theory.

'Coughs and sneezes' do not 'spread diseases'; they spread the *products of disease*, which include the excreted toxins and other exuded emanations of disease and, sometimes, the micro-organisms which find their home therein. This is not to suggest that natural hygiene is unnecessary; indeed, even the sick animal will isolate itself from its fellows. The important point is that the solution to the problem of disease lies in the removal of the causes of the basic ill-health, and not in the avoidance, or the attempted destruction, of the agents of a superimposed infection.

Micro-organisms require food, moisture, a suitable temperature and hydrogen-ion concentration, and, in most cases, oxygen. They will not live long, as a rule, and they certainly will not proliferate, when deprived of these conditions.

The *bacillus influenzae* has lost popularity as the 'cause' of influenza, because the germ is too often frequently found in the throats of people who have no disease, or who have diseases other than influenza, and it is frequently absent in those who are suffering from influenza.

It is now assumed that both influenza and the common cold are caused by a virus. A study of viruses, however, has suggested to some scientific investigators that they are not organisms, but protein-containing enzymes which may be produced within the human body. Certainly they cannot be grown on ordinary laboratory media. They can only be produced from living tissue cells.

For our purpose, enough has been said on this subject; in fact, a deeper study of the various theories and hypotheses can lead only to confusion.

If we now examine some of the various medical methods of treatment it will be clear why they fail.

6.
The Failure of Medicine

THE BRITISH NATUROPATHIC Association of practitioners asserts through its motto, 'Only Nature Cures', that 'treatments' can, at most, provide the conditions necessary for the recovery of health. The naturopath sees his patient as a person with an individual health problem, and he acknowledges the presence of the healing powers that lie within the patient himself. Treatment consists only of removing the obstacles which lie in the way of health, and in aiding the body's natural tendency toward recovery.

Medicine, on the other hand, regards sick people as those who have been 'attacked' by this or that enemy of man. In effect, Medicine says, 'Live as you will; we shall search for a remedy to "fight" all that ails you'. This idea is bound to have a popular appeal but, unfortunately, it does not bring results — at least, not *good* results.

'The war against disease' takes place in laboratories which are completely isolated from the problems of the patient. Clinical medicine, the observation of a patient under the effects of disease, has been relegated to a poor second place behind laboratory investigation. The naturopath contends that the study of human beings in health and disease is the only key to the progress of the healing art, and that the laboratory should be its servant, and not its master.

True health and happiness lie in the growth and development of our *whole* being, and when disorder sets in it is a sign that we have gone wrong somewhere. The work of the consultant should be to seek out the causes of disorder and to advise the sufferer how best he may get back on the road to health. But orthodox medical practitioners are already too busy with their work of prescribing *anti*pyretics, *anti*toxins, *anti*septics, *anti*biotics, *anti*-acids, *anti*spasmodics, drugs to pep you up and others to calm you down, those to tighten a loose bowel, and others to loosen a tight bowel. When medicines fail to remove the *effects* of disease, then surgery may be employed to lop off the offending part or to excise the troublesome organ.

By the suppression of acute eliminative crises the foundation of chronic disease is laid. By relieving ('curing') the patient of the *effects* of disease without removing *causes*, his health goes from bad to worse until the so-called 'incurable' symptoms arise. The source of medical failure is to be found in the notion that 'disease' is an evil thing which 'attacks' the body, and in the belief that somewhere, somehow, an *anti*dote must be found.

For years, the search has gone on for a remedy that would fight the symptoms of 'colds' and 'flu'. Since age-old remedies, like overheating, overfeeding and overworking the body have failed, medical attention has been directed toward *destroying* the invader, or its evil sting. Even though the nature of the supposed invader is still unknown, many poisons are poured or injected into sick people, with the hope that the invader will die but the patient will live. But, alas, to quote a medical writer, 'More than one doctor has treated himself for a simple cold with sulphonamides and penicillin and died as a result'. Even when death or permanent tissue damage does not result from the administration of antibiotics, one or more of many reactions may occur, including nausea, vomiting, glossitis, stomatitis, diarrhoea, skin rashes, etc. — all of which are symptoms of poisoning!

In any case, ill-effect or no ill-effect, in view of our

understanding of disease, it is clear that antibiotics, or any other drug, will not, and cannot, solve the problems of ill-health.

The medical herbalist has his favourite remedies, too, which he claims are non-poisonous. Most of these he considers to be *empiric*, which means that there may be no physiological or pathological reason why they should be used, but that experience has shown that certain results follow their use. In a short article of five hundred words on the subject of 'coughs and colds', a medical herbalist recommends the use of fifty different herbs, and then adds, 'Probably I have missed a few herbs which may be deemed essential by other herbalists, so please understand that the above list is not meant to be exhaustive'. Surely, comment is unnecessary.

To date, all attempts at 'curing' colds and influenza have failed completely, and so attention is now turned to prevention. There are several angles of approach.

It has dawned upon some workers that excessive secretions of mucus (particularly the abnormal discharges of toxaemic persons) form an ideal breeding ground for many of the bacteria that have caused so much medical concern. And so the nasal-douche and the gargle have been reintroduced for the purpose of washing away this excess mucus. (The old idea that antiseptic gargles and douches 'kill the germs of disease' was abandoned long ago.)

Various solutions have been used, mainly expensive and useless antiseptics, but also including salt solutions and soap-suds. Needless to say, this procedure cannot prevent colds, although, if it is carried out frequently throughout life, it may stave off some of the unpleasant sequelae of an over-active mucous membrane. That it has no effect other than the mechanical cleansing of the surface membranes is obvious. The underlying toxaemic condition remains unaffected.

Research on a large scale continues the hunt for a causative virus, with a view to the manufacture of a preventive vaccine.

Recently, the writer had an opportunity to talk with an employee of a well-known firm of vaccine manufacturers. Asked whether or not his laboratories were working on a vaccine for the common cold, he replied that they were not, and added that he did not think that an effective vaccine would ever be made. He then made the surprising statement that he was not in the least worried, anyway, for he had not developed a cold for twenty years. He was persuaded to reveal the secret of his immunity, which was that he had followed the advice of a Nature Cure magazine!

Vaccines do not need to be 'effective' before they are put on the market, however. Several have been on sale for some considerable time, and skilful advertisements maintain sales despite official government announcements that 'it is not at present practicable to consider the development of a vaccine'.

It is easy to supply facts and figures of an encouraging nature concerning the effectiveness of such dubious products. A glance at a table giving the results of immunization against colds — through the use of a widely-used commercial bacterial vaccine — shows that in a group of experimental humans the average number of colds in the year following inoculation was reduced from 4.7 to 2.1. This would seem to be encouraging evidence, until it is discovered that the uninoculated group shows a 6 per cent. greater reduction, namely, from 4.9 to 1.9. The reduction was the result of what has been termed 'the good-and-bad-year phenomenon', and not the inoculations.

Some industrial and business firms have made arrangements for their employees to receive 'immunization' free, or at very low cost. The tremendous response has provided us with adequate evidence that results are very varied. Reports ranged from 'Marvellous', and 'Complete immunity', to 'Hadn't had a cold for many years until I took that stuff', 'Never had a cold like it before in my life', and 'Never again'! It is significant that the initial enthusiasm for this 'free immunity' has now flagged, and in some instances the scheme has been abandoned.

The idea that some sort of 'very wee animal' must be the cause of disease is clung to through thick and thin, and, therefore, the answer is still considered to be a vaccine. It has been 'discovered' that disease can be produced by the injection of putrid fluids into a healthy organism. Severe though it may be, the acute bodily reaction against the introduction of such morbid matter is nothing more than a healthful tissue-cleansing process; but the medical view is that pathogenic (disease-causing) organisms attack the body and result in specific symptoms.

Because the body's efforts to overcome such poisoning include not only elimination but the development of tolerance to poisons, the science of medicine sees fit to promote the development of tolerance, to call it immunity, and thereby forget about removing *causes*.

Instead of building bodily health to the degree where poisoning is dealt with promptly and adequately, 'science' proposes to spare us the discomforts of acute eliminative crises, even though the evil effect of chronic poisoning must inevitably follow. That medicine fails to overcome the chronic diseases also is well known, but that is another story.

7.
The Naturopathic Approach

THOSE WHO SUFFER repeated 'attacks' of the various acute
respiratory diseases that we are considering have usually
suffered also a great many 'treatments' of one sort or
another — doctor's prescriptions, advertised medicines, 'quack'
remedies, and all the 'cures' recommended by friends,
pharmacists and others. None of these does any good, though
some may appear to produce a temporary effect because the
sufferer is forever looking for the smallest glimmer of hope in
the direction of health.

But, slowly, the patient loses heart, and the time comes
when the suggestion that health *is* attainable seems all but
laughable. The idea that a minority movement, known as
Nature Cure, has something better to offer than 'top medical
opinion' appears, to him, truly incredible.

It is this attitude which constitutes the first obstacle on the
road to recovery. Such hopelessness must be broken down.
That is why it is found necessary to expose the fallacy of
medical methods, for once it is clear why symptomatic
treatment fails, then the mind becomes more receptive to a
new approach.

The patient must understand that the common cold is due
to toxaemia, and that the object of Nature Cure treatment is
to get rid of this condition. No 'two-hour cures' are offered;
no pretence is made that a cold can be thrown off like an
unwanted cloak. The purpose of an acute eliminative crisis is
the reduction of a state of toxaemia, and Nature Cure treatments are designed to aid the body's effort in every way possible.
Nature Cure offers *health* — not the mere absence of disease
symptoms, but a condition of physical, mental, emotional,

spiritual and social well-being. This book, however, can no more deal with every aspect of Nature Cure than it can deal with the personal problems of individuals.

Nevertheless, those who put the following suggestions into practice will find that they will not only overcome their tendency to colds, etc., but will feel very much fitter in every way. If further information is desired on this vital subject of health-promotion, a host of published works on all aspects of Nature Cure is available.

THE CRISIS

The violent bodily effort required to bring about an acute eliminative crisis is enervating, obviously. The intensity of the crisis, then, will depend, in part, upon the vitality of the patient. The greater the vitality, the more intense is the crisis likely to be. Patients of low vitality will not, ordinarily, develop a sharp crisis of any intensity, but will be more likely to suffer a series of mild subacute disorders.

It will be noticed that in the young, where vitality is high, acute reactions are (if treated correctly) usually short and sharp, but the enervating habits of modern life gradually reduce vitality until the body can no longer muster sufficient energy for any great exertion.

Therefore, if we forget about 'curing diseases' and think instead in terms of physiological requirements, it becomes clear that the primary need is for conservation of energy in order that the function of the moment (elimination) may be given full play. Usually, though there are exceptions, the body demands this through listlessness, tiredness, and a withdrawal of interest from surroundings, food, etc.

Here, then, is our clue to treatment. The body requires physical and mental rest; and through such rest the body-energy is directed to the job in hand, which will be completed all the sooner if its requirements are understood and provided.

REST, WARMTH, FRESH AIR

Sleep, of course, is the most important form of rest, for during sleep most physical activities are suspended, so enabling the organism to restore vitality and to concentrate on those general maintenance jobs that cannot be undertaken during the hours of activity.

During an acute eliminative crisis as much sleep as possible is desirable, but it must be *genuine* sleep. The state of stupor which is induced by hypnotic drugs is worse than useless, and it would be far better to rest, without sleep. Usually, however, the 'acute case' will have little difficulty in dozing off.

When possible, the patient should retire to bed at the first sign of feverishness and remain there until all the symptoms abate. Occasions do arise when this is impossible, or least impracticable, in which case the patient should do the best he can to obtain the maximum rest possible.

It is important for the body to be protected from chilling, and, in this respect, the patient who is confined to bed is most easily provided for. Night attire should be worn lest the bed-covers be thrown off during sleep. Warmth, however, should not imply a fug. The entry of fresh air into the patient's bedroom is very necessary and, if it be remembered that air currents pass from window to door or fireplace draughts can be avoided easily.

The importance and benefits of fresh air, which has been heavily charged with sunlight and which contains a high proportion of oxygen, cannot be over-estimated. Certainly, the stuff which flows into a window-sealed room from neighbouring rooms (also window-sealed) is no substitute.

FASTING

A large proportion of the energy of the organism is absorbed by the work of digestion, and it is for this reason that the naturopath employs fasting in the treatment of acute disease. When food is not taken this energy is freed, and is devoted to the elimination of toxins.

It is normal and healthful that there should be an aversion to food during acute disease, but this is more commonly observed in animals than in man. One reason for this is that, quite frequently, medical men and well-meaning friends press the patient to 'take something nourishing to keep up the strength'. By coaxing the patient to take a cup of beef-tea a false appetite for other foods may be created, and this leads to the wrong idea that appetite simply needs 'tempting'.

Incidentally, beef-tea contains more toxins, in the form of animal waste-products, than it does nutrients. Even medical men do not now believe in this product as a food. Even should food be 'fancied', we must insist that feeding at this time still further depletes the vitality.

When the alimentary tract is actively engaged in the work of elimination (especially in those cases described as 'gastric flu') much harm may be done by feeding.

If the digestive organs are forced to deal with food when they are busily engaged in eliminating poisons, one of three things must happen:

1. The organs will expend still more energy in throwing off the undesirable foodstuff through vomiting and/or diarrhoea.

2. Elimination will virtually stop to enable digestion to go on.

3. Much of the food will remain undigested in the intestine, where it will ferment and decompose, leading to the formation of noxious gases and other toxic matter. To fulfil physiological requirements, then, we must fast from the time of the onset of symptoms until, at least, the body temperature is normal. This procedure will help shorten the eliminative period.

A fast means abstention from food — all food, that is, with

the sole exception of fruit or vegetable juice. During an acute eliminative crisis an unusual amount of fluid is lost from the body through vomiting, diarrhoea, increased perspiration, etc. In some cases, the organism already has an excess of liquid (which is not at all wholesome) and its loss is a distinct advantage. In other cases, however, particularly where the toxaemic condition is severe, the loss must be made good if elimination is to continue without the patient becoming dehydrated.

Thirst is the finest guide to the body's requirements in this respect. Not the kind of 'thirst' which comes on regularly at 3 p.m. when the tea-cups are rattled, or when the doors of the club bar are opened, but the instinctive desire for fluid which follows a definite deficiency. Excessive quantities of fluid may interfere with the bodily chemistry, particularly the processes of oxidation and elimination.

In the majority of cases, water is without doubt the ideal liquid to take during a fast, but there are two main exceptions.

Firstly, we must consider the quality of the water. Nature provides animal and plant life with water that has been thoroughly aerated and sun-drenched, and is said to be vital to the process of osmosis, which is the basic principle of organic life.

The modern treatment of our mains water not only causes much of the vitality to be lost but, in addition, various chemicals may be added for its alleged improvement or purification or, as in the case of fluoridation, for the purpose of mass-medication. It may then remain stagnant in pipes (often made of lead) for some considerable time before it is used, when further alterations may take place.

Every gardener knows that tap-water is no real substitute for rain, and it requires little imagination to realise that it is not the best water for man. During an acute eliminative crisis the very best materials are necessary if the most thorough job is to be done in the minimum time, and so, if unpolluted stream or rain water is not available, the juice of certain sun-ripened fruits or vegetables is recommended.

In many parts of Britain bottled *Malvern Spring Water* is available, which, apart from filtration, has undergone no processing or adulteration.

The juice of fruits and vegetables is, largely, water, in which is dissolved a quantity of organic substances, of which we are concerned, mainly, with the group commonly known as 'mineral salts'. These help to regulate the flow of fluids to and from the tissue cells in the the process of osmosis, and play many other important rôles. This leads up to our second reason for extracting the water from plants for use as liquid for the person who is ill.

It was mentioned, earlier, that the blood and tissues cannot tolerate an acid condition; in fact, the body is constantly throwing off acid substances in order that an alkaline condition may be maintained. Naturally, the continued supply of alkaline elements is also essential. The tissue-fluids of a toxaemic person carry a too high proportion of acids, which must be eliminated during the eliminative crisis, and we can help to restore balance in this respect if the fluid which we give to the body contains some of the alkaline elements. These important elements include calcium, iron, potassium, sodium, manganese and magnesium, and they are to be found in a great variety of foods, mainly of vegetable origin.

The best juices for our purpose are those which are extracted from any commonly-used green vegetables, including beet-tops, broccoli, etc., celery, root vegetables (especially carrots), and fruits like apples, pears, oranges and tomatoes. It is to be understood that ripeness of the fruits, and freshness of the juices, is of the utmost importance. In some cases, different juices may be mixed to form a sort of cocktail, and it is usually desirable to dilute them with water. Generally, however, it is best if they are used unmixed.

The extraction of the juice is quite a simple matter if a

fruit-juice extractor is used. Without such a useful kitchen appliance, the extraction of vegetable juice, such as from carrots, is best achieved by finely grating the roots and squeezing through a muslin bag. Excellent bottled apple-juice can be obtained from Health Food Stores.

During the period of the fast these juices may be taken as desired, but they should always be sipped and savoured, and not swallowed as a draught.

An essential point to be remembered is that, after a fast (even a short fast of twenty-four hours), the food eaten is absorbed rapidly, and so it must be selected with care. The fast should be broken on fresh fruit, such as apples, pears, peaches, pineapple, etc., and the next two meals, at least, should consist of raw food only. Everything that is eaten must be masticated thoroughly. To summarize, the first few meals after a fast should be arranged as follows: on the day the fast is broken, drink fruit juice on rising. Two or three hours later, take a fruit meal of, say, an apple or two, one or two peaches, or other juicy fruit. At least four hours later, take a small green-leaf and grated vegetable salad with a tomato. A little olive oil or lemon juice is permitted, but no other condiment. The last meal of the day should be of fruit, but a larger quantity may be eaten than was taken for breakfast. On the following day, take fruit juice on rising, fresh or cooked dried fruit for breakfast, a larger salad for lunch, and if desired, a cooked meal in the evening.

Details of the full diet will be given later in the book.

THE BOWELS

In health, the bowels require no attention. When fasting, the digestive organs come to a standstill until food is taken again, and this, in the *healthy* individual, need cause no concern. As the body becomes enervated, or when some other factor causes functional decline of the organs, the retention of waste may add to the troubles of the organism. This is the case, particularly, when the food residue is composed of fermenting and decomposing rubbish which should never have been eaten in the first place, and which, in the second place, was eaten probably at a time when the body was robbed of its appetite because it had no use *for food of any kind*.

During an acute eliminative crisis the organism frequently deals with this situation by the discharge of loose stools, which is known as diarrhoea. When fasting, however, the colon may retain a considerable amount of toxic matter, without which it would be infinitely better off.

The use of purgatives 'to clear the bowels' cannot be permitted by the naturopath, for two main reasons. The action which results from the administration of such medicines consists of a body-effort to eliminate a poison (all purgatives are poisons). This means, of course, that further *enervation* must follow their use and, quite possibly, damage may be done to the delicate mucous membrane of the organs. Also, should the purgative drug be absorbed into the system, acute or chronic systemic poisoning may result. Colonic irrigation is the naturopath's answer to the problem, and, at home, this means using an enema.

A simple enema consists of an injection of nothing but plain water which has been heated to blood temperature (98°F). By means of an injection of between one and two pints, the rectum and lower colon can be cleansed without any damaging effect upon the organism as a whole, or upon the local tissues.

The administration of an enema is simplicity itself. There are two suitable methods:

1. The use of a standard-type enema syringe, by means of which the required amount of water is pumped slowly into the rectum.

2. The use of a douche-can, containing water, which is hung about three or four feet above the level of the patient's

body. An attached rubber tube is greased and inserted into the rectum (about three inches) and, by the release of a stop-cock, the water is allowed to flow in slowly. The patient should be lying on his left side, with knees drawn up. This type of enema may be quite easily self-administered. The retention of the water for a few minutes helps to break up the faecal matter, which is carried away when the water is discharged.

In those cases where the benefit of professional naturo-pathic advice is not available, it is advisable for the patient to use the enema once daily during the fast, after the bowels have ceased to act naturally.

COLD-WATER PACKS

Of the many hydrotherapeutic measures employed in naturopathic practice, the most commonly used in acute disease are the cold-water packs. The full pack and the three-quarter pack are frequent assistants to the naturopath, but they will not be discussed here. The throat-pack, however is very easily applied, and is of great benefit in those cases where considerable congestion of the throat occurs, or where the head feels bloated and heavy. By its action of increasing the local circulation and relieving congestion, much of the discomfort is alleviated and the time-factor involved in tissue-repair is usually reduced considerably. The pack is applied at night and should remain in place until morning.

A strip of cotton or linen material, long enough to surround the neck once or twice (according to the thickness of the material) and about three inches wide, is soaked in plain cold water, wrung out, and applied. This is covered with two or three layers of a slightly wider woollen or flannel material, which is pinned in position with a safety-pin. If the patient is kept warm the pack itself will become warm within a few moments. Only in the case of very devitalized patients will it be found necessary to remove the pack for the reason that no warm reaction sets in.

Whenever the throat-pack is used, a waist-pack should also be applied. The procedure is exactly the same, but the linen should be about eight inches wide, and one thickness is usually enough. The edges must be covered completely by the wider woollen material.

These packs should be used each night during the period of acute distress, but in very many cases, where the full naturopathic treatment is employed, one or two nights will see the end of the symptoms.

The cotton, or linen, material should be washed thoroughly and dried before re-use, and the skin also should be well washed on removal of a pack.

CLEANSING THE SKIN

During acute disease, the skin usually becomes very active in eliminating toxic matter, even when cold packs are not used, and it is desirable that the whole body surface be cleansed of the morbid matter at least once daily during this period. Hot baths can prove enervating, and are not recommended. It is best that the body should be lathered thoroughly with soap and warm water, and rinsed well with a tepid spray. Then rub down briskly with a coarse towel, and return to bed. The operation should be conducted in a warm room, and should be completed within about three or four minutes.

The mucous membrane of the mouth and throat also would benefit from cleansing, which will make the patient feel much fresher. A mouth-wash and gargle of diluted lemon-juice, or salt water (one level teaspoon of salt to a pint of water), is both cleansing and refreshing, but the teeth will usually require cleansing with toothpaste, even when no food is eaten, owing to the sticky nature of the mucus deposits.

MENTAL REFRESHMENT

There is probably nothing quite so enervating as mental and emotional stress. Resentment, frustration, hostility, boredom, etc., will drag down the vitality as quickly as anything, and it is usual for the sufferer to manifest signs of great tiredness. Here, again, we have the common exciting cause, enervation, which precipitates an eliminative crisis.

Some medical workers have noticed that, in certain cases, the development of colds follows immediately some form of emotional stress. They conclude, therefore, that fear, an unsatisfactory sex relation, or some such emotional disturbance may *cause* a cold. But since that conflicts with the opinion that a virus causes colds, an amendment has had to be made.

Medical opinion today holds that there are several different conditions which we call 'colds', differing only in so far as the exciting cause is apparently different. The view taken is that 'at least some outbreaks of colds are due to viruses', but that similar conditions may result from fear or frustration, and a 'cold' was the old-fashioned name given to them all.

Modern medicine is rediscovering the essential unity of mind and body (which means that every thought and every emotion has its effect upon the physical tissues) but by introducing such detailed differential diagnosis the subject is made unnecessarily complicated. We may group together all negative thoughts and emotional stresses and regard them as causative of *enervation*.

The job of overcoming the causes of mental and emotional stress should be left usually until the acute bodily disturbance has passed, for the secret of putting and keeping our emotions in their proper place lies in training and control. For the time being, all that can be done is to relieve the patient of as many enervating influences as possible, by rest, relaxation, and the provision of an atmosphere of pleasant calm. If the patient can be helped to understand, and to trust in, the body's self-cleansing mechanism, a great deal of fretful thinking may be avoided.

At this time, when the body is busily engaged in spring-cleaning, we have an opportunity to excite the mind to a new beginning — a new era of living for health and happiness.

THE TREATMENT OF CHILDREN

It appears that the cold is often the first eliminative crisis to be encountered by a human being; cases are recorded of colds occurring as early as the fourth and fifth day of life. If the causes — toxaemia and enervation — are not removed then, more severe or more frequent crises are likely to follow. The child becomes toxaemic and enervated through the same basic causes as those which influence the adult — faulty diet, chilling, over-tiredness, anxiety, etc., but, usually, the high vitality of the child brings about a quick response, and no lasting or chronic disorder results. If the causes remain, however, then ill-health also remains.

Often, parents try to overcome the tendency to illness by feeding up the child on 'body-builders', vitamin syrups, energy foods and tonics, but, as they fail to remove the causes of ill-health, successful treatment escapes them, and the child is liable constantly to live on the border-line of ill-health. He becomes tired and inattentive, often misses school, and always seems to have a cough or cold, or both.

The constant tiredness leads to a postural droop which, if allowed to persist long enough, will develop into an established postural spinal curvature. This structural defect aggravates the toxaemic condition by interfering with breathing, digestion, and other essential functions. Here, we have the pale-faced, round-shouldered child with his noisy, ineffective cough and his catarrh, and recurrent mild feverish 'attacks' with pallor and headache.

Medical treatments in the form of cough-mixtures, tonics

and 'flu-mixture' can do no good, and some may do slight harm.

In this chapter, we are concerned with the treatment of the 'feverish attacks' and the 'colds', but, in more or less severe cases, the complete restoration of health may require weeks, maybe months, of living in accordance with the principles of Nature Cure, which will be outlined in the following chapter.

At the first sign of an 'attack', protein and starch foods should be withheld, and the sweet and chocolate allowance must be stopped absolutely. The 'luxury' of a day on nothing but delicious, juicy fruit would be of considerable benefit, and if the temperature reaches 101° F, all food should be stopped for twenty-four hours, or until the temperature returns to normal. Hunger disappears at this time, and any plea for 'something to eat' is usually a demand for fuss, rather than food.

On the day following the fast, an all-fruit diet is best. In most cases, it is advisable to have a bowl of mixed, juicy fruits constantly to hand, so that the child knows that quantities are not limited. Appetite alone will then restrict consumption. The fruits most suited at this time are apples, pears, peaches, grapes, pineapple, etc., whereas the highly acid fruits, like plums and oranges, are best avoided until later.

On the second day, after breaking the fast, there should be three meals:

Breakfast. — Fresh fruit, or figs or prunes, cooked with a little honey.

Lunch. — Fruit, and junket or yogurt.

Evening. — A small mixed salad.

On the next day the diet may be increased along the following lines:

Breakfast. — A glass of milk (unpasteurized), given with the fruit.

Lunch. — A cooked meal of poached egg, with spinach or steamed marrow, and a fresh fruit dessert.

Evening. — A mixed salad, with one or two pieces of buttered crispbread. Later, another glass of milk may be given.

Gradually the diet may be increased, more starch and protein foods being included, until the full diet (according to the age of the child) is reached.

Should the skin take part in the eliminative crisis, and the rash of measles develop, the treatment — of rest, warmth, fresh air, fasting, fruit diet, cold water packs, etc. — is exactly the same as for other feverish complaints. All such acute eliminative actions are cleansing and healthful, and they need not be feared if no suppressive treatment is employed.

WHAT THE NATUROPATH CAN DO

Some people prefer to seek professional advice at all times, but as a rule a simple cold, or influenza, may be treated at home without any such help. There are occasions, however, when the severity of the eliminative crisis demands skilled attention, and it would not seem out of place here to mention one or two of the helpful methods employed by the trained naturopath.

The naturopath with an experienced eye will frequently detect the major causes of the patient's disorder, and will marshal his forces toward their speedy removal. He may prescribe the use of full-body packs for the purpose of increasing elimination through the skin, or he may favour some other hydrotherapeutic measure, in any individual case. But his most useful function at this time is, perhaps, the use of his hands in the performance of various manipulative procedures.

As already explained, the damaged and devitalized tissues of a toxaemic individual form an ideal 'soil' for the growth and multiplication of various micro-organisms, and their successful invasion is generally known as infection. Since the toxins produced by such organisms are detrimental to the human body, their rapid proliferation in such 'happy surroundings' may add to the body's already heavy toxic load, and consequently to the work involved in tissue-cleansing. Usually, infection is limited, by the body's protective mechanism, to a local area of devitalized tissue (the respiratory mucosa, in such cases as we are considering here), but, sometimes, bacterial toxins do enter the blood stream, and thereby cause further systemic disturbance. Such a disturbance, however, is, again, action on the part of the body to deal with a poison, and indicates that the patient is responding vigorously to infection.

In some patients the response may be somewhat sluggish, owing to various inhibiting influences which block the vital action of those tissues (widely distributed throughout the body) which normally respond to the presence of such detrimental substances. The naturopath, needless to say, does not seek a *substitute* for vital action, but frees it by the removal of the inhibiting influences.

The manipulative techniques at his command appear to be so easy and simple that the patient, and those around him, are apt to underrate their effectiveness. Each patient is treated according to circumstances and requirements, but the general purpose is to bring about, through vasomotor influences, a movement of the body fluids, affecting every organ and tissue group. This is achieved by the relaxation of contracted muscles, by the establishment of as much spinal articular movement as the patient's condition will allow, and by the correction of spinal lesions. The liver and the spleen are normally very active during acute disease, but in cases of sluggishness, due perhaps to many years of bad posture and shallow breathing, special manipulative measures may be employed to increase the circulation of blood through these organs, which will lead to increased and better function.

It is commonly found that those who suffer disorders of the upper respiratory organs (especially where there are frequent recurrences), sustain many and varied lesions of the vertebral joints of the neck and upper part of the back, and of the surrounding soft tissues. Muscle-spasm, tissue-thickening, joint-fixation and similar lesions frequently result from respiratory disorders and, by interfering with the flow of nerve impulses, may equally well become *causal* factors.

The correction of lesions of this kind may well shorten the period of disease, for, by the restoration of structural integrity, the blood supply, lymph drainage and flow of nerve impulses are freed from restriction, which means more efficient function of the tissues involved in elimination.

Manipulative treatment is of value in most cases of disease and, quite often, it is the quickest of the naturopathic treatments to bring symptomatic relief.

The listed names of practitioners may be obtained from the Registrars of the following organizations:

British Naturopathic and Osteopathic Association, Frazer House, 6 Netherhall Gardens, London NW3.

British Natural Hygiene Society, 91 North Walsham Road, Norwich, NOR 053.

British Register of Naturopaths, 1 Albemarle Road, The Mount, York, YO2 1EN.

SUMMARY OF TREATMENT

One of the great advantages of naturopathic treatment is that there need be no delay whilst diagnostic tests are made. Treatment, which consists of attending to physiological requirements, may commence at the first sign of disorder, and as a result the more severe reactions are often avoided. While the medical man awaits the development of a clinical sign that will clinch the diagnosis before he administers 'specific' treatment, or while medical research workers hunt for an antidote to the virus or viruses that they hope to find causative of colds and influenza, the follower of Nature Cure can help the body to complete recovery by the simple means of aiding toxin elimination.

The exciting cause of acute disease is rather like the straw that breaks the camel's back; it is not of great importance in itself, but on top of the maximum load it becomes intolerable. It is useless to attempt to remove all possible exciting causes with the hope that disease can be avoided, unless the predisposing causes also are dealt with. Recurring eliminative crises indicate that the blood-level of toxins is always dangerously near saturation point and it takes but little to precipitate a crisis. Each crisis reduces the toxaemia to the point of toleration, but unless the causes of toxaemia are removed the balance will swing again in favour of yet another eliminative crisis.

By means of warmth, rest (mental and physical), fastings, cold packs, fresh air, and the judicious use of the enema and manipulative therapy, the body is given every opportunity to eliminate toxins with the minimum of effort. By the avoidance of suppressive medicines the innate intelligence of the body is able to function unhindered, which results in the speediest possible recovery.

In such circumstances the patient is always left in a more healthful physiological condition than he was prior to the crisis.

In the majority of cases, *vigorous* health is not restored even by the naturopathic treatment of acute disease. The toxaemic state is reduced to a safe level, which means that the patient is *healthier*, but the work of building health to a level where there will be no further need for such crises must be done between, and not during, the crises. Depending upon the condition of the patient, such immunity to disease may take from a few weeks to two or three years to achieve, but once attained, it is a treasure to hold.

8.
Building Immunity

IT SHOULD BY now be clear to the reader that the 'curing' of colds is not only unscientific, but very undesirable. The suppression of such cleansing actions can only lead to further bodily damage. If the body cannot free itself of poisonous accumulations, it must store them in the least vital tissues, if it is to survive. Here begins the story of chronic disease development, leading to rheumatism, arthritis, etc.

To achieve immunity from colds our mode of living must be such that *health* is promoted, for there is no magic potion, medical or otherwise, known or sought, that can overcome the ill-effect of living outside of natural law.

The law of cause and effect will see to it inevitably that the degree of health attained is proportionate to the effort put into *living for health*. There is no doubt that, for those who have for years relied upon the medicine-man to overcome their diseases, living for health is an effort, at first. As health is restored — in many cases, such health as has never been known before — the individual finds a new joy in living, and *effort* is no longer required.

Some persons prefer to make changes in their life very slowly, and they naturally, will have to wait longer for the desired result than those who march boldly into a new era of healthful living. But whichever way the change is made, nothing but good can result, and, quite frequently, there are reports of undreamed-of benefits in an almost unbelievably short space of time. Remember, it is not enough merely to wish to be better, or to know how to get better; the mode of living of the sufferer needs to be actively reviewed, revised and reorientated, if he is to be placed on the road to health.

Drastic reform is not always easy for 'friends' are forever ready to point out that one's new efforts are showing no great benefit as yet; they love to point out that weight is being lost, or that a few pimples have developed that were not there before. Determination is necessary to press on, and it is helpful to remember that those who are prolific with directions for the treatment of colds are usually those who suffer such disorders most of all!

Natural immunity (the only *real* immunity) against disease can only be attained if we release ourselves from the many and ever-increasing causes of ill-health. Elucidation on these matters brings with it the possibility of self-help; all that is required then is *action*.

EATING

Many people who turn to Nature Cure for help have already been told by their medical advisers that 'diet' has nothing to do with their disease, and they are surprised when they find that so much emphasis is placed on the subject by the naturopath. It should be borne in mind that naturopaths were insisting on a diet which included *vitamin-containing* raw foods long before 'science' discovered vitamins; that they were using sun-treatmens when the medical-man denied their value; that in medicine, opinions change with the wind, with regard both to the treatment and the prevention of disease.

From the Nature Cure point of view, the same conditions that are required for the recovery of health are also necessary for the maintenance of health. Correct nutrition and efficient elimination are of primary importance. The *quality* of the food eaten should always be considered, the essential qualities being *freshness, ripeness* and *wholeness*.

To obtain the maximum value of the food eaten the process of digestion must be efficient, which means that we should remember that the mouth is not the opening to a waste-shoot; there is a limit to the ill-treatment that the digestive organs can stand. Bad food, combined with the dilution of digestive juices through drinking with meals, the taking of ice-cold or very hot drinks and foods, and over-eating, are some of the very common causes of digestive disturbance.

All foods should be masticated thoroughly and reduced to a pulp, and sloppy foods should be avoided. If these two rules are observed, and no fluid is taken with meals, overeating is unlikely.

AN ALKALINE DIET

By supplying the tissues with a sufficiency of alkaline nutriment, and by keeping the acid-forming foods at a low level, the formation of toxic residues is decreased, and their elimination is facilitated. With but few exceptions the fruits and vegetables constitute the bulk of the alkaline foods, whereas meat, fish and eggs are the main sources of acid-forming foods. The latter are the protein-containing foods, and they are eaten in excess of body requirements by the majority of people.

Because protein foods are very high in calorific value they have been, in the past, considered the most important of all foods. The idea that meat-steaks and strength go together is a popular fallacy of many years' standing, but scientific investigations are proving the naturopathic contention that comparatively small quantities of protein-foods are necessary to the health of a grown adult. In fact, protein need be included in but one meal of the day. To take it with three meals of the day constitutes excess.

The full value of the alkaline fruits and vegetables is

obtained when they are eaten fresh and raw. In this way they give up every essential element they possess, whereas, once they are cooked and processed, much of their value is lost. For this reason, the naturopath recommends that a mixed vegetable salad be taken every day — a practice which will boost considerably the body's alkaline reserve.

Few people would be happy on an entirely raw-food diet, and so the cooking which is done must be designed to cause as little damage to the food as possible. Casserole cookery and steaming are excellent, but the boiling of vegetables does very much more damage and usually results in much of value being thrown down the sink with the water.

The use of soda and salt is condemned, and will be found unnecessary when the more conservative methods of cooking are employed.

Fruits, when cooked, sometimes require a little sweetening and honey or Barbados sugar is recommended for this purpose. White, refined, sugar is taboo. If ripe fruit is selected, little sweetening will be needed.

The starchy foods, also, are often eaten to excess, e.g., bread and porridge at breakfast, potatoes at lunch, perhaps also rice or pastry, bread and cakes for tea, and, at other odd times, biscuits, bananas, etc. To make matters worse, most of such foods are refined e.g., (white flour products and polished rice), which means a loss of valuable vitamins and alkaline mineral salts. The potato, a truly valuable food, is, more often than not, cooked in a manner which causes the loss of its most valuable elements. It should always be cooked in its skin, either baked, steamed or boiled, and the skin should be eaten. If the potato *must* be skinned, it should be done after cooking. Unpolished rice is available at Health Food Stores as, also, are wholewheat flour and bread, and these healthful products should replace completely the devitalized varieties.

Nevertheless, a considerable reduction in the intake of starchy foods is strongly recommended to those who suffer recurrent colds. Naturally, the physically active person will burn more fuel than those who lead a sedentary life, and, therefore, individual requirements will need to be considered. Generally, it may be said that the starchy foods are better confined to two meals of the day or, ideally, to one meal only.

To obtain the maximum benefit from starchy food, its complete digestion is necessary. This process begins in the mouth when the starch particles are ground by the teeth and mixed thoroughly with saliva, which contains the digestive enzyme *ptyalin*. Biscuits soaked in tea, cereals softened with milk, potatoes mashed in gravy, and similar sloppy foods discourage proper mastication and are, therefore, best avoided. Crunchy cereals, toasted wholewheat bread (buttered cold), crispbread and similar hard foods are to be encouraged.

Starch is converted into sugar within the body, and is therefore utilized in the same way as sugar. When starchy foods are included in the diet, adequate sugar is obtainable by the addition of fresh or dried fruits, which comprise the best possible forms of sugar.

The various confections which are included in the average diet impose a burden upon the body processes of oxidation and elimination and require a large amount of alkaline elements for the neutralization of the acids they produce. Advertisements for certain kinds of 'energy foods' suggest that the more sugar one eats the more energy one will have, whereas, in fact, this is untrue. Only the sugar required for work performed will be of value; any in excess of requirements will be a burden, not a boon.

Fats and oils are frequently overeaten, especially by those who suffer from colds, for the supposed purpose of protecting the body from cold. It is true that the layer of subcutaneous fat (just below the skin) serves as an insulator against heat loss, but the consumption of large quantities of fat in the diet in no way promotes health. A small amount of butter, or nut butter, eaten with the daily ration of bread may be considered ample.

Small amounts are also to be had from nuts, and in the form of olive oil as an optional dressing for salads.

For children, one or two glasses of milk may be added daily, but even this is by no means necessary in every case. A drastic cut should be made in the use of fat for cooking purposes, and the frying of foods should be avoided whenever possible. Food prepared with too much fat remains in the stomach for a long time and slows down the process of digestion. Fresh butter and olive oil are the easiest fats to digest.

The acid/alkaline effects of food varies with differences of external conditions in the cultivation and preparation of food, such as the type of soil, the fertilizers and chemicals used, etc. Home-grown fruits and vegetables, from compost-fed soil, constitute the ideal. Some Health Food Stores and green-grocers, in a few towns, sell compost-grown products which carry the guarantee that there has been no contamination with chemical fertilizers or insecticides.

Aside from this, it is important to remember that the fresher the food, the greater its nutritional value; the more processes a food has undergone, and the more additions that are made to it, the less is its true value likely to be.

The present-day consumption of fluids is enormous, and unhealthful. The ideal would be to drink only to quench thirst, and this would be very seldom when the diet is composed very largely of fruits and vegetables. Unfortunately, the drinking of various beverages has become a social habit — almost a social obligation! But, somehow, consumption should be reduced, particularly of the stimulant drinks like tea and coffee. If they *must* be taken *occasionally*, then they should be weak and preferably without milk or sugar. A far better drink would be water or fruit juice.

Never should fluids be taken with meals, for the simple reason that digestion is upset through the dilution of the digestive ferments.

The use of condiments and strong spices is to be discouraged. Very often they are used to disguise spoiled or adulterated foods, or to stimulate an unnatural appetite. The majority of them have little or no food value. It is common knowledge that the effect of spices, peppers, etc., is due to their irritant action upon the mucous membranes of the stomach and intestines, but it is not generally realized that the same irritant action is at work on the membranes of the upper respiratory organs, resulting in an increased mucus secretion of the nose and throat. Chocolate will often have a similar irritant effect.

There is, of course, no objection to the use of such herb flavourings as mint, marjoram, thyme, parsley, chives, etc.

ARRANGING MEALS

Definite rules about the method of arranging meals cannot be laid down to suit everyone. The health of the individual, his hours of work, the nature of the work, and whether or not all meals will be available at home will have to be considered in each case.

A specimen dietary may be outlined for general guidance, but adjustments of one sort or another will be necessary in many cases. Readers who would like further information on food combining, and healthful daily menus and recipes, are referred to the excellent books on these subjects published in this series.

The customary three meals a day may be continued conveniently, and if the need is felt for a little refreshment between meals, one of the juicy fruits is best, say, a peach, a pear, or an apple.

Many people have no desire for food on rising from bed, and for them breakfast is best omitted. Fresh fruit makes an ideal breakfast for those who desire it, and, for variety, fresh and dried fruits may be taken together as a fruit salad. In winter, when there may be a desire for a little more food, toasted wholewheat bread or a wholegrain breakfast cereal may supplement the fruit.

A daily salad (to provide vitamins, alkaline elements and other invaluable organic substances) may be eaten at midday or in the evening, whichever is most convenient. It should consist of a good variety of green-leaf vegetables such as cress, watercress, lettuce, or chopped cabbage or Brussels sprouts, with tomato, beetroot, celery, cucumber, radishes, etc., as available. One lettuce leaf and a slice of ham is *not* a salad! A little fresh lemon juice or olive oil may be used as a dressing. A small amount of grated cheese, or a portion of cottage cheese, and a slice or two of buttered wholewheat bread or crispbread completes the meal.

The third meal of the day may be cooked one — unless enthusiasm creates a desire for another salad, in which case the bread should be replaced by a portion of protein food, such as cheese, egg, beans, peas or nuts.

The cooked meal should include potatoes (cooked as described previously), one or two green or yellow vegetables, and a savoury dish of protein food. If meat is to be included in the diet, then it should form part of this meal, but the less often it is eaten the better. For dessert, fresh or cooked fruit, or an occasional egg custard is suggested.

When there is no desire for food, a meal should be missed. (The body will benefit from this digestive rest, which should be thwarted by snacks of tea and biscuits or other 'pickings'). Even when appetite is good, an occasional rest from food will help those who are trying to build immunity to colds. One day, every other week, without food of any kind, or a couple of days each week without breakfast, or some similar restriction is often advantageous.

At the first sign of a cold, forego all food and apply treatment as described in the previous chapter. After the fast, increase the diet slowly, starting with the fruit and vegetable juices, followed by the raw foods, and eventually adding the cooked foods.

SKIN TONE

A healthy, active skin is necessary if we are to secure immunity from colds, for two main reasons. Firstly, because only a healthy skin can serve as an efficient eliminator of toxins, and, secondly, because we depend upon the activity of the skin for the capacity to react to changes of external temperature. It is important that the body should be capable of dissipating excessive heat, and to be able to retain body heat when the external temperature is low.

Normally, the skin reacts to heat, cold, light and touch (which includes friction and pressure), and these stimulants keep the skin healthily active. Unfortunately, modern civilized living tends to protect the skin in many ways, so that much of its tone is lost.

The same stimulants are all that is necessary for the restoration of good tone. Light may be provided by periodic exposure to direct sunlight of the whole, or part, of the body, or by the exposure to daylight, if not sunlight, as often as possible, and by the wearing of clothes which permit light rays to reach the body surface, at least in part.

Most skins are continually overheated by clothing or overwarm room atmospheres, and so exposure to cold is the required stimulus. Hot baths are best avoided for this reason; a comfortably warm bath should be followed by a quick, cold shower. It should be noted, however, that the cold shower is merely a means of promoting better skin tone; it does not in itself *protect* the body from colds. Frail types should not scorn warm water with the idea that resistance to colds will follow a spartan existence. A feeling of warmth and comfort should quickly follow the use of the cold shower; if it does not, then the cold water should be withheld for a while, until better powers of reaction have been developed.

Skin friction, by rubbing the body with the palms of the hands has a useful stimulant action, and the effect may be intensified by the use of a dry, coarse towel. The combined effect of friction and cold may be obtained through a vigorous rub-down with a towel that has been wrung out of cold water. This may be followed by the dry friction rub.

Even exposure of the skin to the air is of some benefit, and this can easily be done whilst washing or doing other jobs before dressing in the morning. Slapping the skin is a very invigorating practice which may conveniently become part of the after-toilet procedure.

Clothing should be light in weight, and loose. Air should be able to circulate over the body surface without hindrance from clinging, restrictive garments. Cellular materials are probably the most comfortable to wear, and they are certainly the most hygienic. Irritant materials, and those which prevent the speedy evaporation of perspiration, are not healthful. Overheating the body is not a good thing whether it be due to faulty dress, overheated rooms, too many bed-covers, or sitting in the hearth. A skin which is overheated for long periods will soon lose its tone.

The skin and mucous membranes are complementary; what affects one affects the other. By increasing the tone of the skin, the mucous membranes are relieved of much eliminative work, but a flow of mucus, to a small degree, is essential to keep the mucous membrane healthily moist. Centrally-heated atmospheres, and those heated by gas or electricity, frequently become too dry, and this tends to dry out the mucous membranes of the respiratory tract. In such circumstances it is best to try to preserve a degree of humidity in the air by allowing a bowl of water to vaporize in the room.

The mouth-breathing habit, if present, must be overcome, for it causes the air passages to become too dry. The nose is especially equipped to moisten, warm and filter air before it is passed to the lungs.

THE BOWELS

With the recommended dietary in full use, few people will have trouble with bowel action, with the result that no purgative medicines are necessary and the intestinal mucosa will develop a healthy tone. In some cases, bowel sluggishness is the result of muscular atony, and abdominal exercises are necessary for the restoration of healthy muscle. Good posture, particularly in the walking and sitting positions, is essential to proper muscle usage, and so should be cultivated to the exclusion of bad postural habits. Most abdominal exercises may be combined with breathing exercises, for the muscles of the abdomen and thorax work in unison. The ability to use the lungs to the full is of great importance to the processes of oxidation and elimination.

Any of the conventional exercises are suitable, including body rotation, side-bending, stretching, and forward and backward bending, while breathing continues steadily and rhythmically.

One very useful exercise for the abdomen is simple retraction, which may be performed inconspicuously at any time and in any good postural position. Without causing any chest movement, the abdominal wall should be drawn in as far as possible, and then relaxed. Those with very much weakened muscles may need to assist the movement at first by the use of the hands. Practised occasionally throughout the day, this exercise will increase the tone of the muscles of the abdomen as well as those of the intestine, and, of course, it stimulates the circulation of blood throughout the organs of digestion and elimination.

The best all-round exercise, without a doubt, is walking. When performed in a good relaxed posture, it benefits the whole body. The muscular movements help to increase the general circulation of blood, and provide a truly natural massage to the organs of the abdomen. Such healthful muscular exercise will bring about a complete combustion of the energy foods, and the elimination of simple waste products is facilitated by the increased heat production. A keener appetite, and better digestion and assimilation, are the inevitable result.

Most types of sport are useful as forms of physical exercise, but it should be remembered that it is healthful to exercise only long enough to produce a state of tiredness. It is unwise to become exhausted. Here lies the greatest danger of competitive sports — everyone is trying to outdo everyone else.

THE INFLUENCE OF THE MIND

It is not realized sufficiently that bodily functions are influenced profoundly by every change of mood, and that the power of thought may modify these functions. Although everyone has heard of cases where severe fright has turned hair white in a night, few people seem to realise the depressing nature of stresses of a lesser degree.

One of the most common causes of nervous maladaptation is lack of constructive outlet for the utilization of surplus energy. An outlet is required primarily as a form of expression of the personality, but it should be designed also to provide a great amount of pleasure to the individual. The desirability of congenial employment is obvious, but even where this is impossible the development of a pleasurable hobby can provide the required gratification. In most cases, however, if a person truly hates his work, and never takes a pride in it, it would be worth almost any sacrifice to look for a different kind of work. Enervation results far too easily from discontent, disharmony and discord.

It must be remembered that thought, aided by the imagination, may predetermine pleasurable or unpleasurable experiences. For example. ice-cold water may feel scalding-hot to the hands if one believes mistakenly that it flows from a hot-water tap. The temperature of swimming pool water always seems more comfortable to those who look forward with great pleasure to their swim, and a similar expectation often predetermines the extent of one's pleasure in visiting a theatre.

The same attitude of expectation, in which thought plays so great a part, causes remarkable repercussions in all avenues of life and is a powerful predetermining factor in effecting the final issue. If we fail to see anything of interest in our work, we may be sure that our work will not offer us any interest. If we cultivate the art of using the imagination for the purpose of creating clear mental images of our desired achievements in life, we can become thoroughly familiar with every aspect of the ideal, and, by so doing, set for ourselves a pattern, or mould, after which one's life may shape itself. By creating new mental paths for the will to travel, we can direct our life activities along new channels, and, with tenacity of purpose, anything may be achieved.

The adoption of the Nature Cure way of living is made easy by such means, provided that one does not stop at the half-way house of the imagination — the day-dream. Those who remain content with the work of mental pattern-making will achieve nothing. Dreams must be made real to be of any value. We all tend to act according to our old feelings and desires, but the will must be directed along the new paths at all times, if success is to be achieved.

Once the decision is made to act upon naturopathic advice, no side-tracking should be allowed. Stick to the decision through thick and thin, until well-beaten mental paths have been formed.

Mental fatigue may create the impression that such efforts are not worth while, and if such fatigue develops readily in spite of the adoption of the physical treatments outlined in this book, it is to the mind that one should look for the cause.

Resentments, frustrations, inner conflicts and boredom are common causes of mental tiredness, and these troubles will need to be faced squarely if fitness is to be achieved.

Conclusion

EVERYBODY DESIRES TO know 'How long will it take to develop a high degree of health and an immunity to colds?' Naturally, the answer will depend upon one's physical condition at the outset. A great many people come to Nature Cure after many years of drug treatments, and they consider the 'new' method to be merely 'worth a last try for health'.

It may take two years, or more, to rebuild such an ill-treated body into a healthy condition, but nature is usually kind and health is restored very much more quickly than this.

In some cases, colds disappear completely as soon as the new way of life is adopted; in others, a few sharp eliminative crises may follow in rapid succession before the toxaemic condition is cleared.

We must not lose sight of the fact that an eliminative crisis is a *healthful* action on the part of the organism, and that, in itself, it does not constitute ill-health. Without such eliminative efforts, toxaemia could mount to a fatal level, and, therefore, we should not be distressed if our bodies have an occasional spring-clean.

Immunity from colds can never be guaranteed absolutely, for the simple reason that modern man is exposed continually to new, detrimental influences, which tend to produce toxaemia and/or enervation. 'Science' invents new methods of preserving foods, of making stale foods taste fresh, and of colouring and flavouring in many ways. New, artificial substances are being produced in the guise of food and medicine. Drinking water is doctored, the atmosphere is polluted, atomic radiations increase, and various medical concoctions, such as vaccines, are pressed upon an innocent public.

But the Nature Cure movement is alive to the situation, and a constant watch is kept on these new developments. The public is informed of the possible dangers, and how they may be overcome, through the British Naturopathic and Osteopathic Association's publications. The reader would be advised to keep abreast of the world's health news through these channels.

A long continued toxaemic condition induces a certain degree of toleration to toxic matter, and a super-saturation of the blood may develop before a crisis occurs. When health is built up, however, and the system is cleansed of morbid matter, a lesser degree of toxaemia will bring about an acute eliminative reaction. This quick response ensures that the tissues never become chronically poisoned, and, therefore, chronic diseases, so-called, do not occur.

The prevention of colds, then, depends upon the maintenance of a healthy blood stream — a condition enjoyed by the many thousands who follow Nature Cure.

Those who wish to join the ranks of the physically fit should remember that there is no time like the present — for *action*.